FAST TRACK DIET FOR LPR

20 Fast relieving recipes to heal lpr, gerd and acid reflux quickly

CELINE BAMAS

TABLE OF CONTENTS

15. Veggie Omelette with Mushrooms and Spinach

16. Baked Tilapia with Roasted Brussels Sprouts

17. Apple and Walnut Salad

18. Carrot and Ginger Juice

19. Chicken Caesar Salad with Low-Fat Dressing

20. Pumpkin and Chia Seed Pudding

1. Grilled Chicken with Steamed Vegetables

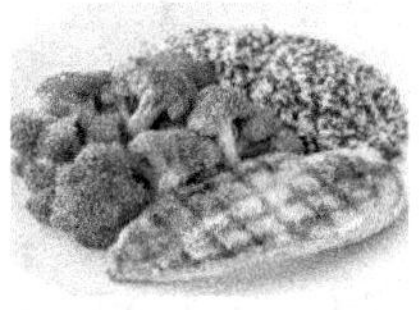

Ingredients:

- 2 boneless, skinless chicken breasts

- 1 cup broccoli florets

- 1 cup carrots, sliced

- 1 cup green beans

- Olive oil

- Salt and pepper to taste

Instructions:

1. Season the chicken breasts with salt, pepper, and a drizzle of olive oil.

2. Preheat the grill to medium-high heat.

3. Grill the chicken for about 6-8 minutes per side or until cooked through.

4. Steam the vegetables until tender, about 5-7 minutes.

5. Serve the grilled chicken with steamed vegetables.

Caloric Information (Approximate):

- Grilled Chicken: 165 calories per 3 oz (without skin)

- Steamed Vegetables: Varies based on portion size

2. Baked Salmon with Asparagus

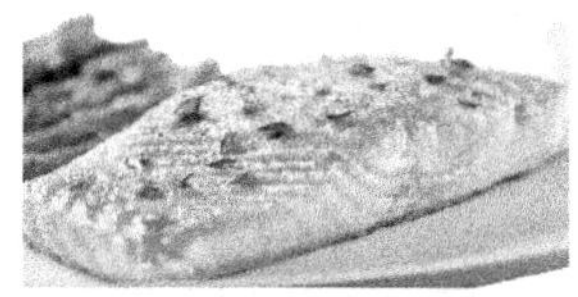

Ingredients:

- 2 salmon fillets

- 1 bunch of asparagus

- Olive oil

- Lemon juice

- Salt and pepper to taste

Instructions:

1. Preheat the oven to 375°F (190°C).

2. Place salmon fillets and asparagus on a baking sheet.

3. Drizzle with olive oil and lemon juice. Season with salt and pepper.

4. Bake for 12-15 minutes or until salmon flakes easily with a fork.

5. Serve with lemon wedges.

Caloric Information (Approximate):

- Baked Salmon: 367 calories per 6 oz fillet

- Asparagus: 20 calories per cup

3.Avocado and Spinach Smoothie

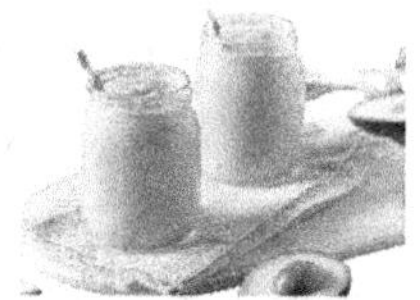

Ingredients:

- 1 ripe avocado

- 1 cup spinach leaves

- 1 banana

- 1 cup almond milk

- Honey or sweetener (optional)

Instructions:

1. Blend avocado, spinach, banana, and almond milk until smooth.

2. Add honey or sweetener if desired.

3. Serve immediately.

Caloric Information (Approximate):

- Avocado: 234 calories per avocado

- Spinach: 7 calories per cup

- Banana: 105 calories per medium banana

- Almond Milk: 30-40 calories per cup (unsweetened)

4. Quinoa and Roasted Vegetable Salad

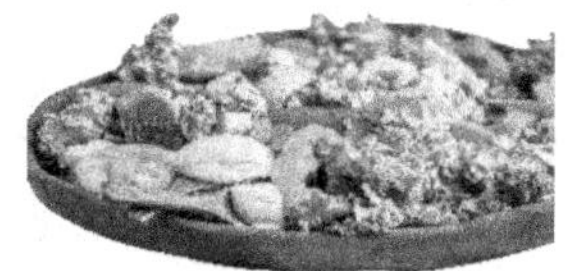

Ingredients:

- 1 cup quinoa

- Assorted roasted vegetables (e.g., bell peppers, zucchini, cherry tomatoes)

- Olive oil

- Balsamic vinegar

- Fresh basil leaves

- Salt and pepper to taste

Instructions:

1. Cook quinoa according to package instructions and let it cool.

2. Toss roasted vegetables in olive oil and roast until tender.

3. In a bowl, combine quinoa, roasted vegetables, fresh basil, olive oil, balsamic vinegar, salt, and pepper.

4. Serve chilled.

Caloric Information (Approximate):

- Quinoa: 222 calories per cup (cooked)

- Roasted Vegetables: Varies based on selection

5. Turkey and Sweet Potato Stew

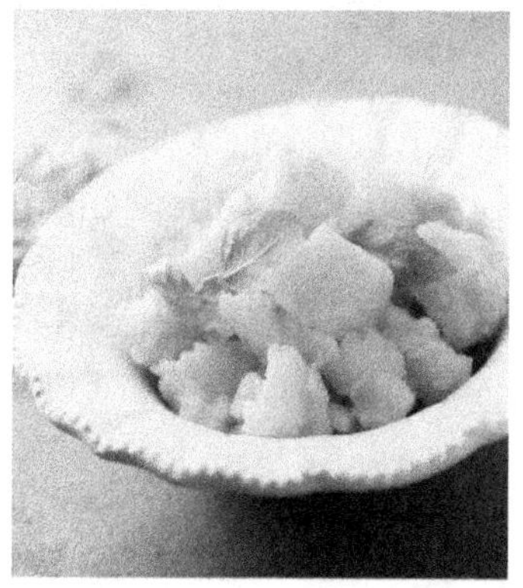

Ingredients:

- 1 lb ground turkey

- 2 sweet potatoes, diced

- 1 onion, chopped

- 2 cloves garlic, minced

- 1 can diced tomatoes

- Chicken broth

- Spices (e.g., paprika, cumin, chili powder)

- Salt and pepper to taste

Instructions:

1. In a pot, sauté onions and garlic until fragrant.

2. Add ground turkey and cook until browned.

3. Add sweet potatoes, diced tomatoes, and spices.

4. Pour in enough chicken broth to cover the ingredients.

5. Simmer until sweet potatoes are tender.

Caloric Information (Approximate):

- Ground Turkey: 211 calories per 4 oz (cooked)

- Sweet Potatoes: 180 calories per cup (cooked)

- Other ingredients: Calories vary

6. Zucchini Noodles with Pesto

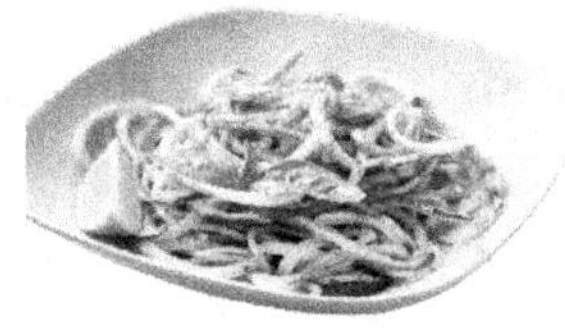

Ingredients:

- Zucchini noodles (zoodles)

- Pesto sauce

- Cherry tomatoes, halved

- Parmesan cheese (optional)

Instructions:

1. Spiralize zucchini into noodles.

2. Toss zoodles with pesto sauce and cherry tomatoes.

3. Optionally, sprinkle with Parmesan cheese.

Caloric Information (Approximate):

- Zucchini: 20 calories per cup (raw)

- Pesto sauce: 80-100 calories per 2 tbsp

- Cherry tomatoes: 27 calories per cup

7. Baked Cod with Lemon and Dill

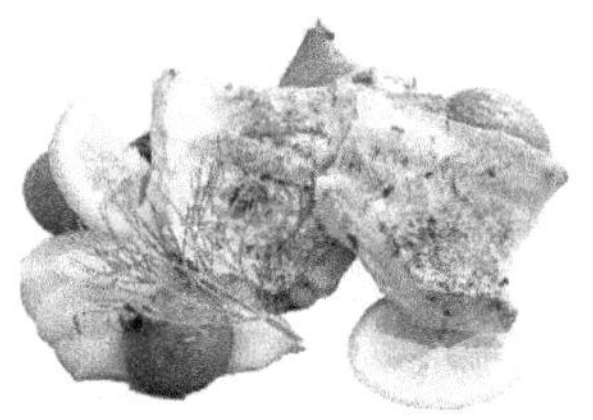

Ingredients:

- Cod fillets

- Lemon juice

- Fresh dill

- Garlic powder

- Salt and pepper to taste

Instructions:

1. Preheat the oven to 375°F (190°C).

2. Place cod fillets on a baking sheet.

3. Drizzle with lemon juice, sprinkle with fresh dill, garlic powder, salt, and pepper.

4. Bake for 15-20 minutes or until fish flakes easily.

Caloric Information (Approximate):

- Cod: 105 calories per 3 oz fillet

8. Lentil Soup with Carrots and Celery

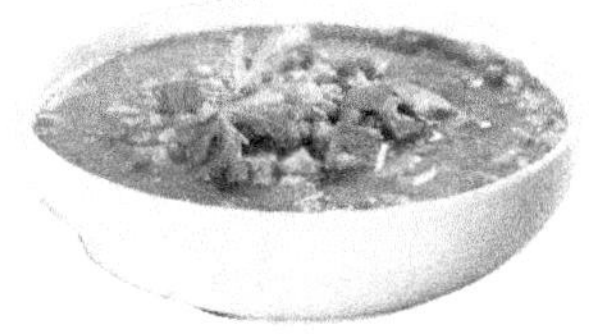

Ingredients:

- 1 cup dried lentils

- Carrots, chopped

- Celery, chopped

- Onion, chopped

- Vegetable broth

- Spices (e.g., cumin, coriander, turmeric)

- Salt and pepper to taste

Instructions:

1. Rinse lentils and place them in a pot with chopped vegetables and vegetable broth.

2. Add spices and seasonings.

3. Simmer until lentils and vegetables are tender.

Caloric Information (Approximate):

- Lentils: 230 calories per cup (cooked)

- Other ingredients: Calories vary

9. Cauliflower Rice Stir-Fry

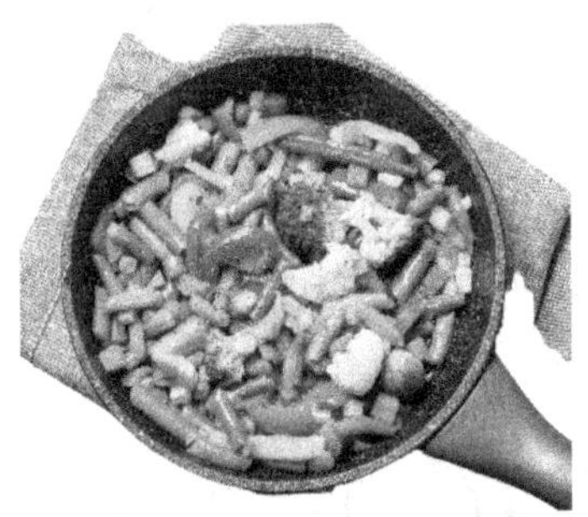

Ingredients:

- Cauliflower rice

- Mixed vegetables (e.g., bell peppers, peas, carrots)

- Tofu or chicken (optional)

- Soy sauce

- Sesame oil

- Garlic and ginger (minced)

- Green onions

Instructions:

1. Sauté garlic and ginger in sesame oil.

2. Add cauliflower rice, mixed vegetables, and protein (if desired).

3. Stir-fry until cooked through, adding soy sauce for flavor.

4. Garnish with green onions.

Caloric Information (Approximate):

- Cauliflower Rice: 25 calories per cup (cooked)

- Other ingredients: Calories vary

10. Almond Butter and Banana Oatmeal

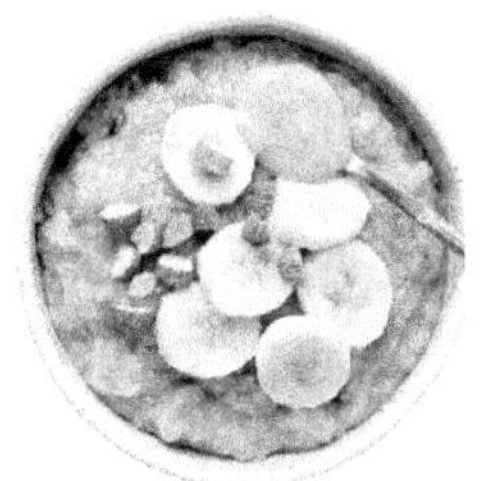

Ingredients:

- Rolled oats

- Almond butter

- Banana, sliced

- Honey or maple syrup (optional)

Instructions:

1. Cook rolled oats according to package instructions.

2. Stir in almond butter and banana slices.

3. Drizzle with honey or maple syrup if desired.

Caloric Information (Approximate):

- Rolled Oats: 150 calories per cup (cooked)

- Almond Butter: 98 calories per tablespoon

- Banana: 105 calories per medium banana

- Honey or Maple Syrup: Calories vary

11. Poached Eggs with Sautéed Spinach

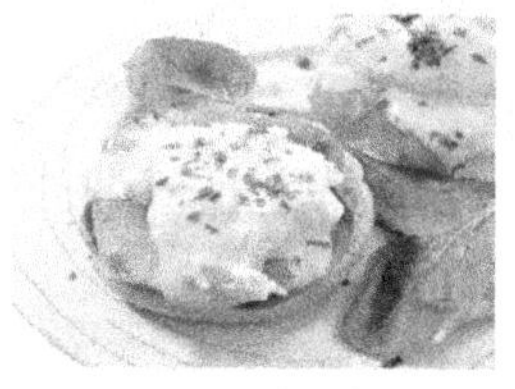

Ingredients:

- 2 large eggs

- 2 cups fresh spinach

- 1 teaspoon olive oil

- Salt and pepper to taste

Instructions:

1. Heat olive oil in a skillet over medium heat.

2. Add fresh spinach and sauté until wilted, about 2 minutes.

3. Fill a saucepan with water and bring it to a simmer.

4. Crack the eggs into separate cups.

5. Carefully slide the eggs into the simmering water.

6. Poach the eggs for about 3-4 minutes for a runny yolk, or longer if desired.

7. Remove the poached eggs with a slotted spoon and place them on top of the sautéed spinach.

8. Season with salt and pepper.

9. Serve immediately.

Caloric Information: Approximately 220-250 calories.

12. Grilled Tofu with Broccoli

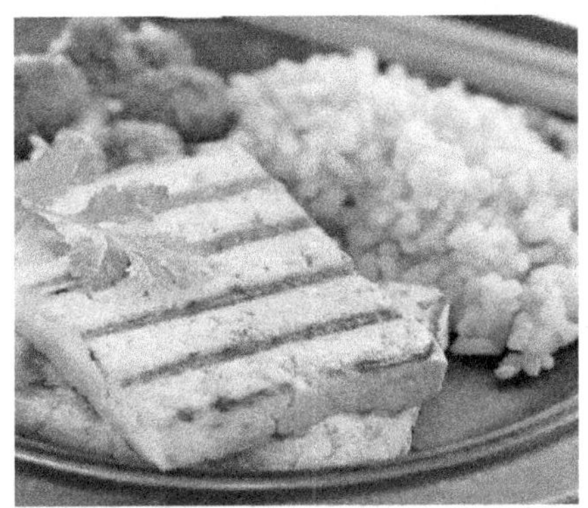

Ingredients:

- 8 ounces firm tofu

- 2 cups broccoli florets

- 1 tablespoon soy sauce

- 1 teaspoon olive oil

- 1/2 teaspoon garlic powder

- Salt and pepper to taste

Instructions:

1. Press the tofu to remove excess moisture and cut it into cubes.

2. In a bowl, mix soy sauce, olive oil, garlic powder, salt, and pepper.

3. Marinate tofu cubes in the mixture for 15 minutes.

4. Preheat a grill or grill pan over medium-high heat.

5. Grill tofu and broccoli for 5-7 minutes, turning occasionally until grill marks appear.

6. Serve hot.

Caloric Information: Approximately 250-280 calories.

13. Roasted Butternut Squash Soup

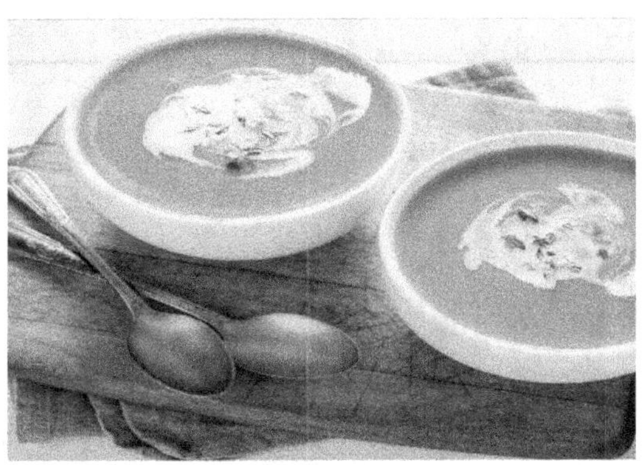

Ingredients:

- 1 medium butternut squash, peeled and cubed

- 1 onion, chopped

- 2 cloves garlic, minced

- 4 cups vegetable broth

- 1 teaspoon olive oil

- Salt and pepper to taste

- 1/2 teaspoon ground cinnamon

- 1/4 teaspoon nutmeg

- 1/4 cup heavy cream (optional)

Instructions:

1. Preheat the oven to 400°F (200°C).

2. Toss butternut squash cubes with olive oil, salt, pepper, and ground cinnamon.

3. Roast in the oven for 25-30 minutes until tender.

4. In a large pot, sauté chopped onions and garlic until translucent.

5. Add roasted butternut squash and vegetable broth. Simmer for 10 minutes.

6. Use an immersion blender to puree the soup until smooth.

7. Season with nutmeg and add heavy cream if desired.

8. Simmer for an additional 5 minutes.

9. Serve hot.

Caloric Information: Approximately 150-180 calories (without heavy cream).

14. Greek Yogurt with Berries and Nuts

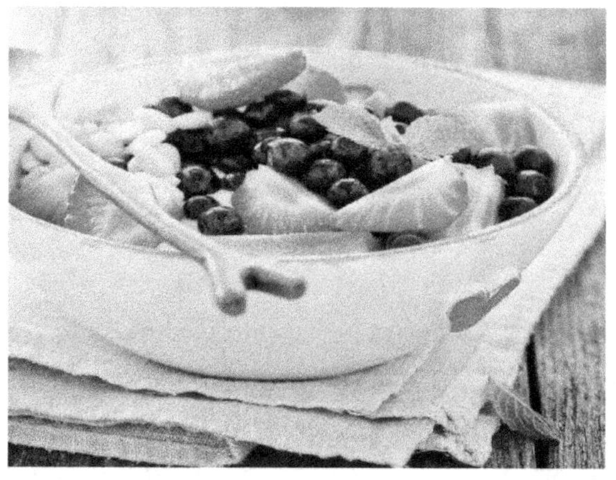

Ingredients:

- 1 cup Greek yogurt

- 1/2 cup mixed berries (e.g., blueberries, strawberries)

- 1 tablespoon chopped nuts (e.g., almonds, walnuts)

- Honey or maple syrup for drizzling (optional)

Instructions:

1. Spoon Greek yogurt into a bowl.

2. Top with mixed berries and chopped nuts.

3. Drizzle with honey or maple syrup if desired.

4. Serve as a healthy breakfast or snack.

Caloric Information: Approximately 180-220 calories (without sweetener).

15. Veggie Omelette with Mushrooms and Spinach

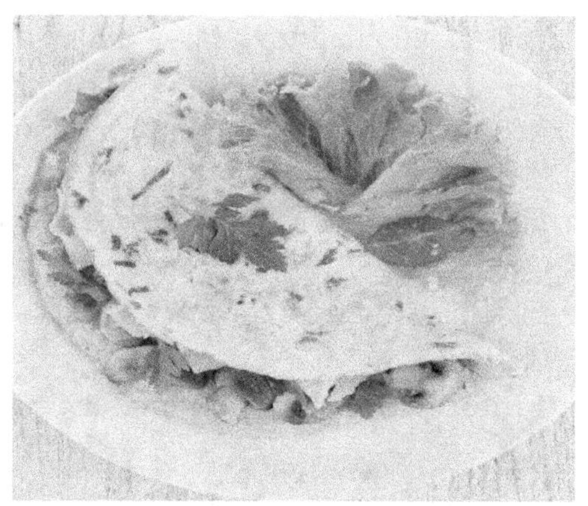

Ingredients:

- 2 large eggs

- 1/4 cup sliced mushrooms

- 1/2 cup fresh spinach leaves

- 1/4 cup diced bell peppers

- Salt and pepper to taste

- 1 teaspoon olive oil

Instructions:

1. Heat olive oil in a non-stick skillet over medium heat.

2. Add mushrooms and bell peppers, sauté for 2 minutes.

3. Add fresh spinach leaves and sauté until wilted.

4. Beat eggs in a bowl, season with salt and pepper.

5. Pour beaten eggs over the sautéed vegetables.

6. Cook until the edges set, then flip and cook the other side.

7. Serve hot.

Caloric Information: Approximately 200-230 calories.

16. Baked Tilapia with Roasted Brussels Sprouts

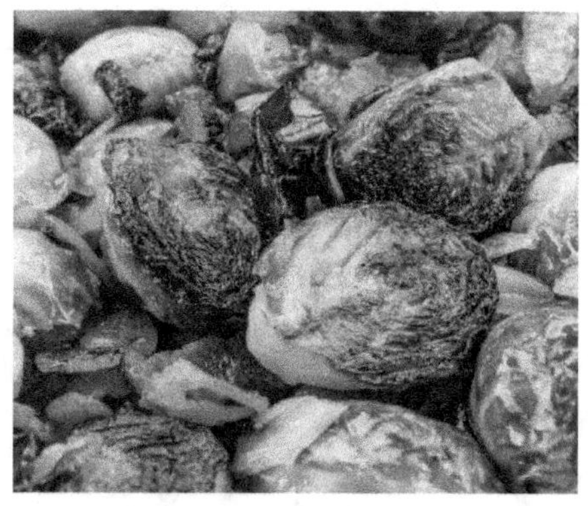

Ingredients:

- 2 tilapia fillets

- 2 cups Brussels sprouts, halved

- 1 tablespoon olive oil

- 1 teaspoon lemon juice

- 1/2 teaspoon garlic powder

- Salt and pepper to taste

Instructions:

1. Preheat the oven to 400°F (200°C).

2. Toss Brussels sprouts with olive oil, lemon juice, garlic powder, salt, and pepper.

3. Place tilapia fillets on a baking sheet and season with salt and pepper.

4. Arrange Brussels sprouts around the tilapia.

5. Bake in the oven for 15-20 minutes until fish flakes easily.

6. Serve hot.

Caloric Information: Approximately 250-280 calories.

17. Apple and Walnut Salad

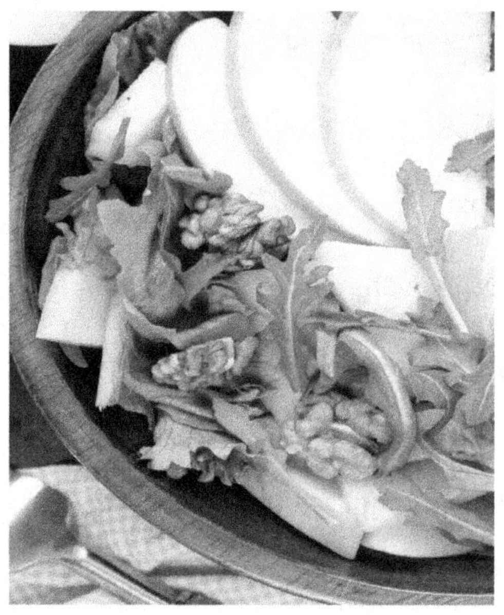

Ingredients:

- 2 cups mixed salad greens

- 1 apple, thinly sliced

- 1/4 cup chopped walnuts

- 2 tablespoons balsamic vinaigrette dressing

Instructions:

1. Toss mixed salad greens with sliced apples.

2. Sprinkle chopped walnuts over the salad.

3. Drizzle with balsamic vinaigrette dressing.

4. Toss to combine.

5. Serve as a refreshing salad.

Caloric Information: Approximately 220-250 calories.

18. Carrot and Ginger Juice

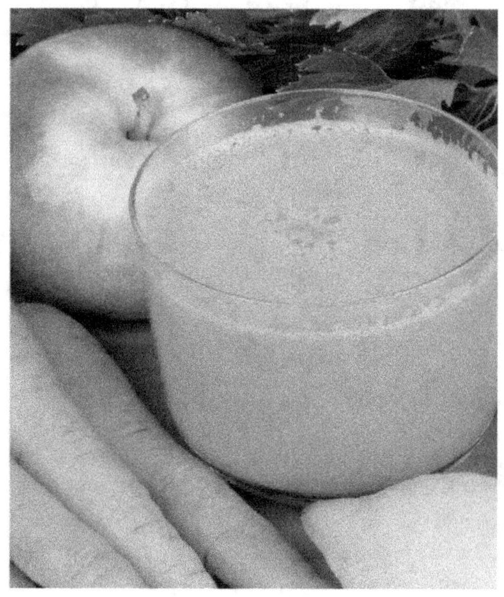

Ingredients:

- 4 large carrots, peeled and chopped

- 1-inch piece of ginger, peeled

- 1/2 lemon, peeled

- Water (as needed)

Instructions:

1. Run carrots, ginger, and lemon through a juicer.

2. Add water to adjust the consistency if needed.

3. Serve as a nutritious juice.

Caloric Information: Approximately 120-150 calories.

19. Chicken Caesar Salad with Low-Fat Dressing

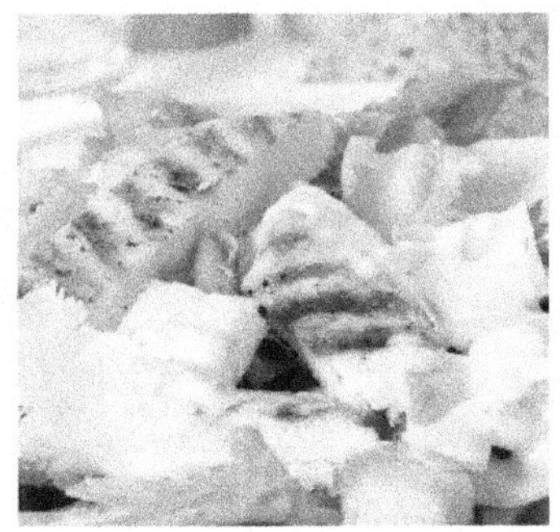

Ingredients:

- 4 cups romaine lettuce, chopped

- 1 grilled chicken breast, sliced

- 2 tablespoons low-fat Caesar dressing

- 1/4 cup croutons

Instructions:

1. Toss romaine lettuce with grilled chicken slices.

2. Drizzle low-fat Caesar dressing over the salad.

3. Sprinkle croutons on top.

4. Serve as a satisfying salad.

Caloric Information: Approximately 300-330 calories.

20. Pumpkin and Chia Seed Pudding

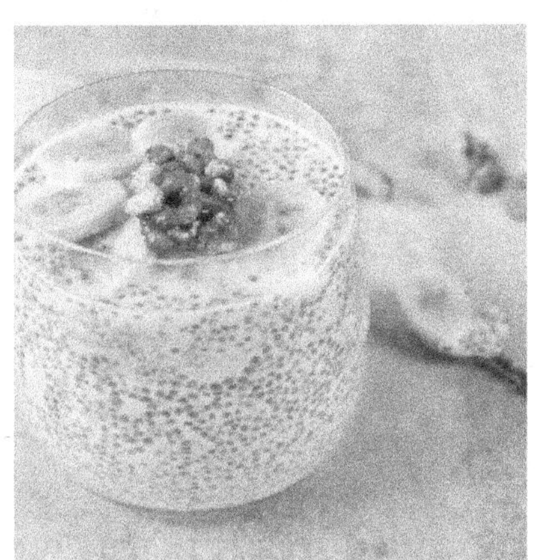

Ingredients:

- 1/2 cup canned pumpkin puree

- 2 tablespoons chia seeds

- 1/2 cup almond milk

- 1 tablespoon maple syrup

- 1/2 teaspoon pumpkin pie spice

Instructions:

1. In a bowl, mix pumpkin puree, chia seeds, almond milk, maple syrup, and pumpkin pie spice.

2. Refrigerate for at least 2 hours or overnight to thicken.

3. Serve as a delicious pudding.

Caloric Information: Approximately 180-210 calories.

CONCLUSION

Dear valued readers and supporters,

I wanted to take a moment to express my sincere gratitude to each and every one of you who purchased my LPR Diet Cookbook. Your support means the world to me, and I'm truly touched by your decision to embark on this journey to better health with my recipes.

I hope that the cookbook has not only provided you with delicious and nutritious meal options but has also been a source of inspiration on your path to managing LPR effectively. Your commitment to your well-being is admirable, and I believe that with dedication and the right choices, you can achieve your health goals.

Wishing you all the best on your LPR Diet journey. May each meal you prepare from the cookbook bring you comfort and nourishment. Remember that taking care of yourself is a beautiful act of self-love, and you are making positive strides towards a healthier and happier life.

If you ever have any questions, feedback, or simply want to share your culinary adventures, please don't hesitate to reach out. Your stories and experiences inspire me to continue creating and sharing recipes that support your health and well-being.

Thank you once again for your trust and support. Here's to your health and happiness!

Warm regards...